The Fit Arthritic:

Fighting Knee and Hip Arthritis with Exercise.

ALAN KELTON M.D.

Photos and Illustrations:
Nicholas Lopez
www.conceptsbynicholaslopez.com

First published by Dog Ear Publishing
4010 W. 86th Street, Ste H
Indianapolis, IN 46268
www.dogearpublishing.net

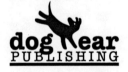

dog ear
PUBLISHING

ISBN: 978-1598585-620-6

This book is printed on acid-free paper.

Printed in the United States of America

To Susan, from you I gain strength.

Contents

Foreword

I dream of running. When the dreams start, I am running in a rolling meadow. I can feel the breeze on my face. I feel euphoric, in a runner's high. It seems easy to pace up a hill and then cruise down the slope with long smooth strides, my legs easily handling the weight of my body as the slope approaches level ground. I find myself surprised by the easy motion in my knees and the feeling of exhilaration, while thinking that there should be over-powering pain and stiffness. Abruptly, I then wake after a few moments of this bittersweet, recurrent dream.

It has been about 25 years since I have been able to run. I was 19 when I had my first injury to a knee (the second knee had hidden damage that was revealed in surgery 12 years later.) I reluctantly gave up competitive volleyball and took up bicycling as a way to rehabilitate the one damaged knee. A few years later, I had to give up cycling when my damaged knee would give out then swell unpredictably on hard rides. My other knee, the good knee, now itself has had classic osteoarthritis for more than 10 years.

Before my knees were damaged, I used to tease friends about their weight loss diets as I had always been able to exercise to any weight I desired without any worry over food. I even maintained a slim 175lbs on my 6 foot 2 inch frame when I cycled in my early 20's, eating ice cream almost every day. I was once told by a college athlete that I was the most fit person he knew at that time. Unfortunately, the recovery after my first surgery did not last. I did not have a long term plan for fitness and joint protection and I did many things that sabotaged my mobility. Over time, sadly, my weight ballooned to 240-plus blubbery pounds due to the combination of painful knees, a typical American diet and lack of exercise. I was obese and in pain daily from my arthritic knees.

More than 10 years later, in medical school, my knees were a teaching resource for my classmates with their uneven range of motion, crunch and crackle "crepitance" with movement and the swelling that would arise with a few minutes of activity.

I am now in my mid-forties and pleasantly enjoying mostly pain-free days. I used to consume more than 2000 ibuprofen tablets yearly and now I rarely take them for knee pain. I can walk for extended distances and finished a day-long hike in Yosemite National Park this year. I am finally back at a healthy weight around 175 pounds. I have discovered many principles that have helped me to become more active, suffer from less pain, and yes, consider myself fit once again.

Interestingly, these principles were not emphasized by the doctors who cared for me. General physicians truly do not have the time to teach us how to care for our joints nor do many know what to teach. Orthopedists (doctors who operate on bones and joints) are paid to operate, and are also too busy to help us care for ourselves. For most doctors their interest is in what to do for today's pain, not what to do for tomorrow's mobility.

This book is a reference primarily for those with hip or knee arthritis as these joints are commonly affected and tend to limit aerobic activity such as walking, jogging, cycling or dance. Lack of aerobic exercise contributes to weight gain, heart disease and unfortunately, worsening arthritis.

Osteoarthritis is a common disease and you may know that you have it before reading this book. I, however, discourage self-diagnosis and treatment without input from a specialist in osteoarthritis. Osteoarthritis and your joints may change over time requiring changes in activity or treatment. I encourage you to take information from this book and share your fitness goals with your doctor, physical therapist, sports medicine doctor or orthopedic surgeon. Encourage them to help you evaluate your present level of fitness and progress in achieving good health.

My hope is that you will find what you need to start or maintain an exercise program and achieve the best level of fitness so that you may also consider yourself a "fit arthritic."

Achieving Fitness

Fitness, with osteoarthritis (OA), is the optimum combination of strength and cardiovascular health with maintained mobility.

The pain of OA keeps most of us from exercising. Just the thought of exercising can bring out aches in our affected joints. Typically, pain is nature's way of saying "stop doing that." Avoiding pain is good, usually. However, the saying "No pain No gain" may actually apply to OA. There will be pain with or without exercise and starting a new exercise routine may cause more discomfort at the outset. I believe, however, that for most of us a good exercise program will reduce pain while promoting health.

Personally, I have given up on being as fit as I was 25 years ago. I cannot run, nor can I spend hours cycling as I have in the past. This loss of joint function had been discouraging and had kept me from pursuing fitness and health for my arthritic body. In recent years, I have changed my attitude and adjusted my fitness goals to attainable and satisfying ones for my own health and longevity. This required me to enjoy memories of my more fit past, but not try to relive it. I finally forgave myself for 70 pounds of weight gain and the worsening of my OA because of the weight gain. With my new goals and attitude, I have gradually increased my exercise so that I am more fit than just 10 years ago. Weight loss has helped decrease the amount of pain and stress my knees used to feel. I can now walk for miles on flat ground. I can walk stairs most days when in past years, working in the hospital, I had to choose the elevator more often than I wanted. My long term goal now is to have maintained mobility (walking, primarily) without joint replacement. I want to be able to walk my grandchildren to school. I want to be able to ballroom dance with my wife when we are retired. I no longer want to return to running, or to be able to cycle over 100 miles in a day. I do not regret being unable to push or move heavy weight with my previously strong legs. Unfortunately, I still cannot go near a volleyball game without joining in, and if I do, I am limping and in pain for weeks afterward.

My experience has verified personally what the medical literature supports. Exercise for our damaged joints helps minimize the pain and disability that we experience. It is, however, true that excess or heavy exercise may damage our joints or initiate OA. Excess joint stress can hasten our need for joint replacement. But what are we to do? Just waiting for joint replacement is not a good option. Many with OA will gain weight by avoiding activity and thereby risk heart disease, diabetes and suffer from other weight-related conditions, including worsening OA. Besides, most with OA who have joint replacements do not lose weight and the mobility gained by artificial joints tends not to allow brisk exercise.

I am confident that exercise is one of the factors that may stabilize OA and prevent or slow progression. Exercise may therefore delay or prevent joint replacement. Besides, a joint replacement, if inevitable, is better faced by a fit patient with a strong and supple leg. So forgive yourself for any health problems you may have caused and then make a plan to start living in a healthy way. A key to healthy living with or without OA is exercise.

I recommend that you exercise almost every day. Start with a few minutes of activity and slowly increase over time. Five minutes of walking, cycling or other aerobic exercise is a good start. Start two to three days a week. As your confidence builds, exercise again for five minutes at a different point of the day. Add more five or ten minute episodes over time. It is a reasonable long term goal to exercise 30 minutes most days of the week. Yet, on the days when exercise seems too difficult consider spending a few minutes with strengthening exercises, such as seated leg-lifts for OA of the knees, or by exercising other areas of the body if your achy joints won't allow their use. It is ok to take time off. I recommend having one day off per week to avoid burnout (boredom) and to allow your muscles and other soft tissues to relax and repair. You may also want to have a way to allow one or two "joint relief" days per month in which you allow yourself partial or complete relief of exercise activities.

Expand your definition of exercise. Once you can move your body in a walking or cycling program consider adding other activities to your exercise program. Dance, especially ballroom or square dance, would be a wonderful way to add low impact movement to your activities. Swimming or pool exercise is wonderful for OA and obesity. Yoga, Tai Chi and other forms of traditional exercise are valid forms of exercise for those of us with OA. Add walking to your errands, this increase your overall time in exercise. Parking centrally and walking to multiple stores will help or parking in the spot with the best shade and the most distant from the store will also help.

It is important to have fitness goals. Ultimately, it may be difficult to have a goal of just being able to exercise for 30 minutes. It is better to have the goal of walking your grandchildren to school, for example. Or, like me, plan a hike that you may have had to miss in the past. Maybe graduating from a wheelchair to a walker or cane while in the grocery store may be your goal. The way to achieve the goal is to gain the strength and the cardiovascular endurance to do so.

Fitness, the combination of strength and cardiovascular health with maintained mobility, can be both a goal and a reward. Less pain and increased mobility is what most of us want right away. These rewards are easily recognized and measured and once you have them you will not want to give them up. Improved cardiovascular health decreases your risk of heart attack, stroke and dementia. It also lessens the chance that you will be dependent on others. Mobility is a key to independence and allows for more possibilities in shopping and leisure activities whether alone or with others.

I am trying to live up to the definition of fitness for OA. I exercise most days. I am active up to 30 minutes or more on most days. I exercise my weak and diseased joints and enjoy training and using the joints that are not adversely affected. I give myself time off and use some "joint relief" days. My short term goal of walking with my family to our favorite pancake house every week came easier than I had thought. My long term goal of performing an all-day hike with my wife (a hike I last did 24 years ago, a year after my first knee surgery) was achieved last summer as part of our 20th wedding anniversary.

To summarize, you do need to exercise, even with OA. You may also need to change your definition of exercise to include other activities within your capacity. Start two to three times a week five minutes at a time. Add five minute routines in at later parts of the day. Move not just your affected joints, but also other parts of your body. Plan to have one day off per week even after your fitness goals are attained. Have alternate activities available for the days in which your joints will not allow typical exercise. Give yourself some "joint relief" days off, as long as you keep to your goal of improved overall health. Find a way to measure your success and have multiple goals for your improved body to enjoy. With these principles I am confident that you can become a "fit arthritic" and enjoy improved cardiovascular endurance, a stronger body and greater mobility.

Osteoarthritis: The Pain and the Stiffness

Osteoarthritis (OA) is a common joint disorder in which the joint surface wears away resulting in pain, stiffness, abnormal joint growth and intermittent swelling. Normal joint surface is made up of a type of cartilage, articular cartilage. Healthy articular cartilage is mostly water. There are cartilage cells, and other molecules that hold the water tightly in the joint surface. The articular cartilage is naturally very smooth and absorbs some of the energy from the impact of joint use. Damaged joint surfaces absorb less energy and are more likely to be damaged by jarring or heavy weight bearing. The joint fluid is also affected by OA and becomes less lubricating than normal joint fluid. Exercise, such as running, in healthy joints does not necessarily cause "wear and tear arthritis" as the old expression had indicated. Injury, obesity, inherited joint mechanics and heavy joint loads in sports or work may all contribute to the development and the rate of joint wear in OA.

The symptoms of OA are pain and stiffness. The stiffness is classically noted in the morning or when starting movement such as getting out of a car after a long drive, or arising from sitting. The stiffness lasts less than 30 minutes, and most of us experience just moments of stiffness early in the disease. The pain in arthritis can be mild and momentary or can be deep, aching and debilitating. The pain along with the stiffness may disappear during activity or exercise and then return after stopping or may return with prolonged activity. Interestingly the pain from OA does not come from the worn joint surface. The joint surface itself has no pain receptors and cannot send pain messages to the brain or spinal cord. The surrounding tissue (capsule) around the joint has many pain receptors as does the bone on either side of the joint. It is from the capsule and the bone that the pain signals arise. Sometimes the pain actually arises from the hollow center in the bone marrow. This may be why pain from the hip can be felt in the knee or pain in the knee from the thigh to the calf.

The pain receptors around the joint cause reflex relaxation of the muscles that support the joint. This contributes to muscle weakness and wasting, which can then contribute to increased joint wear. The reflex weakness may also show up episodically. When a person with hip or knee OA arises from a chair or uses stairs they will sometimes experience a sensation of sudden collapse. This reflex "give way" sensation is similar to dropping a hot pan. Pain from the joint tissue is transmitted through nerves to the spinal cord and the spinal cord reflex causes muscles to relax, before we are aware of either the pain or the reflexive weakness. Fear of pain and fear of "give way" collapse often preclude us from performing otherwise safe and helpful activities. This is where self knowledge and education comes to play. Review the exercises and pain diagrams in this book often to develop and maintain awareness of your arthritic joints.

Nature's way of saying "stop doing that" is pain. We learn early in life that we are happier when we do not injure the sensitive areas of our bodies. This tendency to avoid pain is still good, but the fear of pain in OA keeps us from being healthy. Good health requires at least two things from us. We need to eat well and exercise. If we do not exercise we cannot have good health as the risks of heart disease, obesity, and osteoporosis are only some of the problems that increase with time and inactivity.

It should be noted that OA is typically not a problem of severe swelling. It is not a disease associated with fevers, weight loss, red or hot joints or skin changes. The stiffness sensation lasts almost never longer than 30 minutes. If these other symptoms are present most physicians would undertake analysis of blood and joint fluid, along with x-rays to find an explanation and initiate treatment for something that is not likely to be OA.

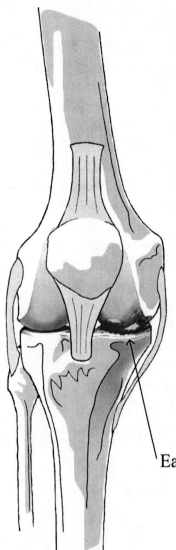

Osteoarthritis, as in the illustration starts with a small amount of damage to the articular surface cartilage. Microscopic damage later gives way to visible damage and loss of cartilage volume. The volume loss is seen on x-rays as the bones becoming closer together. "Bone on bone" arthritis is when most of the articular cartilage has been lost. The meniscus cartilage is often damaged prior to the articular surface degeneration. The meniscus can also be damaged by the irregular bony growth that can occur from osteoarthritis.

Early Medial Joint Arthritis

Get a diagnosis

Osteoarthritis is an easy disease to diagnose. Pain and stiffness of an affected joint that arises after rest or inactivity and that is relieved within 30 minutes of activity without any other outstanding symptoms or features is most likely OA. There are, however, many joint disorders that may mimic OA that are better treated by specialists or with special medications or approaches. A good physician will rely on your story of the symptoms along with an exam and possibly with X-ray or other diagnostic techniques to verify the diagnosis. Get your diagnosis now so that you can get on with your life and achieve your best fitness while maintaining mobility.

X-rays are important in the evaluation of arthritis. They can verify the typical findings of OA. Sometimes they may point to a cause of the arthritis. For example, joint misalignment may be best seen and measured on X-ray. Additionally, findings may demonstrate cartilage calcification that may prompt your physician to look for metabolic diseases such as gout and hemochromatosis (excess iron, a common inherited condition.) If findings of rheumatoid arthritis are found on X-ray, especially if unexpected, you would want your condition evaluated by a rheumatologist (a rheumatologist is a physician specialist in autoimmune and arthritic conditions).

Early in the disease, an x-ray may appear and be interpreted as normal. This does not eliminate the diagnosis of OA. OA is a disease affecting the articular cartilage, and articular cartilage is invisible on x-ray. An MRI may show the changes in the cartilage, but besides being an expensive test, MRI would not usually help in the diagnosis or treatment of OA. Remember too, that neither x-ray nor MRI helps to diagnose pain. A person may have advanced arthritis on x-ray yet may report little discomfort or immobility. Severe pain, alternatively, may not be reflected in either image test but MRI should be considered when pain or worsening symptoms do not fit typical OA.

Laboratory analysis of joint fluid, especially if joint swelling is present, should be considered. Evaluation of inflammation, and possibly of autoimmune tests by blood analysis may also be considered if the diagnosis of osteoarthritis is in doubt. If you have had hot or red joints at anytime, a thorough exam, lab analysis and x-ray panel should be undertaken. Hot and red joints essentially rule-out osteoarthritis. The one possible exception to this rule is osteoarthritis that develops after a gout attack. In this circumstance gout should be treated and the joints cared for as if the primary joint disorder is osteoarthritis. Gout is a common, often inherited, condition in which the joints become red, severely painful and swollen due to crystals of uric acid forming in the fluid of the affected joint. Gout typically attacks the feet and legs. There are sometimes fevers with gout and astute physicians may consider joint infection as a possible alternate explanation to gout symptoms. Interestingly, gout may attack previously damaged joints of a person with OA.

I want to emphasize my concern that you get a diagnosis. There may be an underlying and treatable condition that when found and treated, may improve your joint condition. It is especially important that if your joints are stiff for more than 30 minutes, swell frequently, are ever hot to touch, are red, or have any association with fevers, sweats, weight loss, intestinal symptoms or rash that you have your doctor do a complete examination to find the cause of your symptoms. Osteoarthritis is a non-inflammatory condition of one to multiple joints characterized by stiffness, pain, joint enlargement and sometimes fluid swelling. Conditions other than OA may be treated like OA if the underlying condition is treated or inactive. The diagnosis of OA is usually straightforward, but just to be safe I want you to have your physician diagnose the condition, and ultimately agree with your plan to take care of your joints and your health.

The Pain and its Treatment

OA gives us a variety of pain. There is the stiffness and sudden pain of first movements. There are also the deep bony aches that can linger and keep us from sleeping. There may be swelling and capsular pain that is worsened by fully extending or bending the joint. And sometimes there is more.

A damaged joint has lost its balance. The fine structural associations of healthy joints give way to laxity or stressed ligaments, tendons and other structures. Tendonitis may be more common in our damaged joints. Tendonitis is the inflammation of the part of our muscle that attaches to the bone; it is an achy to burning sensation associated with movement of the joint and is usually tender to touch. Closely associated is bursitis. Bursitis is the inflammation (pain) of the fluid filled flat sacs that separate moving tissues. Touch your elbow and wiggle the skin at the tip of the elbow. The easy movement of your skin is due to a bursa, a part of your body of which most are unaware, unless it has been injured. The knee has multiple bursae (plural of bursa). Sometimes the searing hot and pinpoint pain in or around that arises from nowhere and disappears in hours or days may be one of the multiple bursae, suddenly inflamed, that surround your joint.

It is important to track your pain. As with my case, I believe that successful joint care reduces overall pain, even if at times it seems to temporarily make the pain worse. Keep a journal of pain and function using the letters PSS (pain, stiffness and swelling) and compare it to goals of fitness to keep you on track to improved health. Please keep in mind that severe and deep pain, especially if persistent, may need further investigation, even if your initial diagnosis with your physician revealed typical OA.

Use my diagram to help assess your pain. Compare them to the diagnoses from your physician. You may be able to manage your pain if you know that, for example, the severe pain that seemed to hobble you this morning is simply a small and generally harmless case of bursitis.

Treatments for pain

There are multiple treatments for the pain of osteoarthritis. There are topical therapies such as heat, ice and topical rubs. There are also TENS devices (transcutaneous electrical nerve stimulation), acupuncture and massage. Most topical therapies, including acupuncture, work by distracting your brain and spinal cord from the pain or by blocking the pain signal at the spinal cord. None of these therapies change the process of OA. Ice, I believe, is best used when recent swelling or injury occurs, not for routine or daily pain management.   This is especially true for OA as pain and stiffness seem to be enhanced by cold joints or cold weather. Topical treatments have the advantage of lack of interaction with other essential medications. An OA sufferer may try multiple types of topical therapy without having to check with a doctor regarding possible side effects or medication interactions. Use some caution as a salicylate (aspirin-like) containing topical agent was recently linked to a young athlete's death when high doses of the cream and patches were used. I am intrigued by capsaicin, a chemical derived from peppers. Topical use of a capsaicin treatment can deplete the spinal cord of a key pain relay substance, substance P, stopping the flow of pain signals from the area in which capsaicin is applied. You may want to try one the capsaicin containing creams if you can tolerate a couple of days of burning sensation the creams create.

There are oral medications for OA. Most of us are aware of acetaminophen as in Tylenol, ibuprofen as in Advil or Motrin and naproxen as in Aleve. Aspirin, ibuprofen and naproxen are in a class of medications called NSAIDS (non-steroidal anti-inflammatory drugs). Acetaminophen is unique and unrelated in its mechanism of pain control compared to the NSAIDS. In general, the NSAIDS are better at pain reduction in OA than is acetaminophen. For many, however, acetaminophen may be safer. The NSAID type medicines have risks of hypertension, reduced kidney function, bleeding or stomach ulcer bleeding. Ulcer bleeding risk increases

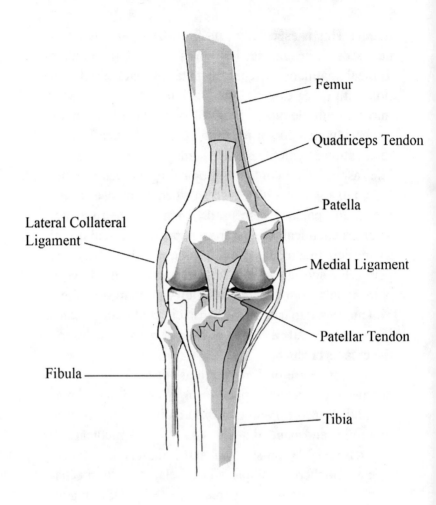

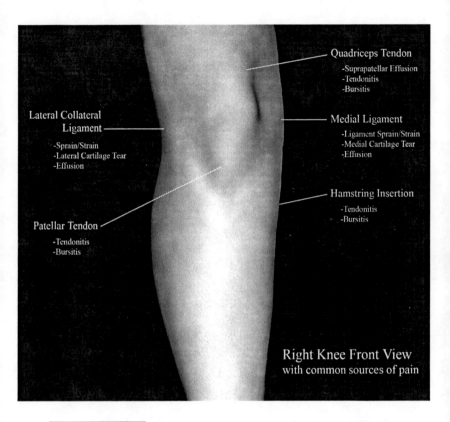

Right Knee Front View
with common sources of pain

Quadriceps Tendon
-Suprapatellar Effusion
-Tendonitis
-Bursitis

Medial Ligament
-Ligament Sprain/Strain
-Medial Cartilage Tear
-Effusion

Hamstring Insertion
-Tendonitis
-Bursitis

Lateral Collateral Ligament
-Sprain/Strain
-Lateral Cartilage Tear
-Effusion

Patellar Tendon
-Tendonitis
-Bursitis

Use these diagrams to better understand your knee structure and possible sources of pain.   Please touch your joint structures so that you can recognize where they are and how they may contribute to discomfort in an arthritic joint.

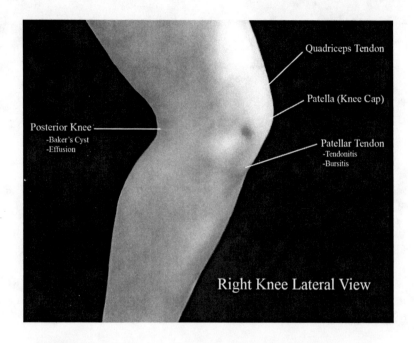

Quadriceps Tendon

Patella (Knee Cap)

Posterior Knee
-Baker's Cyst
-Effusion

Patellar Tendon
-Tendonitis
-Bursitis

Right Knee Lateral View

Not all sources of pain are included in these illustrations. Arthritic joints often ache deeply and diffusely, especially if the pain is coming from the bone or marrow space. Knowing what a particular point of pain is, or why it arises may help to deal with localized pain.

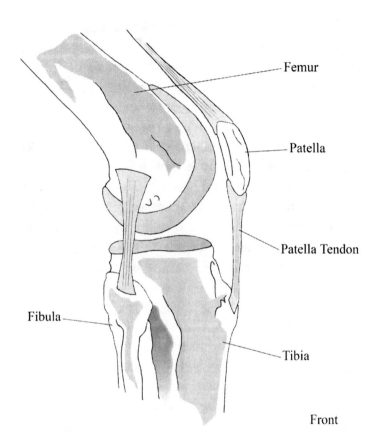

Femur

Patella

Patella Tendon

Fibula

Tibia

Front

with age, and if occurs may be life threatening. There is a class of newer medications, the COX-2 inhibitors, Celebrex is the remaining example. The others, Bextra and Vioxx, have been removed from the market. The COX-2 inhibitor, Celebrex works like an NSAID, but when used alone has a decreased risk of stomach ulceration when compared to other NSAIDS. Most NSAIDS will interfere with aspirin if aspirin is used to prevent stroke or heart attack, and NSAIDS increase the risk of stomach ulcers when used with aspirin. None of these medications are completely safe, including acetaminophen, and these medications should not be taken daily. Acetaminophen may itself be associated with liver and kidney failure especially when taken continually, at high doses or with the use of alcohol-containing beverages. The use of these medications should be coordinated with your physician and the benefit of intermittent, frequent or daily use should be weighed against the risks these medicines may pose for you. Please also keep in mind, none of these medicines change the disease process of OA. A topical NSAID has recently been approved for use with osteoarthritis of joints of the upper or lower body. In short-term use it does not appear to have the same risks as an oral NSAID. Check with your medical professional to see if you may benefit from this new preparation.

Opioid medications (medications that are similar in structure or function to morphine) may offer relief for those with severe and persistent pain. Opiates are typically well tolerated, not toxic though with prolonged use may lead to some immune system suppression or decrease of sex hormone levels. In overdose, these medications may result in death due to cessation of breathing. These medications may also be very addictive. There is some concern for toxicity of the combination acetaminophen and opiate combinations (such as Tylenol #3, Vicodin, Lortab, Norco, Percocet and many others). These opiate/acetaminophen tablets may be toxic in that some people will take too much of the acetaminophen component chasing a "high" with the opiate or adjusting the dose without awareness of the risk of these medications. Most of these medications will cause constipation and prophylactic use of stool softeners or laxatives to maintain normal bowel movements is required. Again, opiates or opiate combinations do not change the disease process of OA and are best used intermittently, except in severe persistent pain.

So far, the use of medications as described above may be different than you may have thought. All of them have some risks and none of these medications change the course of your OA. If they help you to stay functional, to improve your strength and cardiovascular health and help you participate in essential activity the medicines are being wisely used. If you take them reflexively or on a schedule, you may want to try stopping the medication. I used to take more than 2000 ibuprofen tablets a year early in my course of OA, and I would take handfuls of aspirin to compete in volleyball tournaments. I am fortunate that I did not suffer from any serious side effects of the medications.

What about supplements? Supplements may have a role as part of OA treatment. Please remember that there are no cures for osteoarthritis, regardless of what you have heard or read. The use of glucosamine, for now, may have some merit. There are numerous studies using glucosamine or glucosamine and chondroitin in OA. The most recent, the GAIT trial, published in the New England Journal of Medicine February 23, 2006 seems to show no benefit at six months of therapy for mild osteoarthritis. There may be, based on this study, reason to think that those of us with moderate to severe disease or fluid swelling (effusion) may benefit from glucosamine/chondroitin, however. If you would like to try the supplement, buy a brand that has independent quality review and does not exceed your comfort for cost. Most forms of glucosamine are derived from shellfish so avoid them if you have shellfish allergy. If in 3-6 months you notice no effect, stop the medication and see if there is a difference after stopping. Similarly, fish oil, especially if being taken for cholesterol management or cardiovascular disease risk reduction may be tried for joint pain relief. Fish oil supplements reduce inflammation and this may then reduce joint pain. There are many other supplements that are promoted to improve joint function, none of which have enough scientific evidence to be included in this edition.

There are other medications being evaluated for OA including doxycycline (an antibiotic) and others that are being tried in animals. It is not reasonable to recommend these or other new agents at this point. It is quite likely that if we could compare the available medications to the combination of healthy exercise and weight loss that the healthy habits would be far superior to the effect of any current medication or supplement. Please don't buy into the hype, there is no cure and there is no medication or supplement that returns your joint to a more youthful state. Start with topical treatments, consider glucosamine and chondroitin and then use the other medicines intermittently as tools to help you become a fit arthritic. Please check with a physician knowledgeable about the benefits and potential toxicities of these treatments to determine what, if any, medications or supplements you may take. Good activity and a healthy diet may be all you need to become a "fit arthritic" with me.

Level of:		Sunday	Monday	Tuesday	Wednesday	Thursday	Friday	Saturday	Total Score
Week 1	Pain								
	Stiffness								
	Swelling								
	Fitness								
Week 2	Pain								
	Stiffness								
	Swelling								
	Fitness								
Week 3	Pain								
	Stiffness								
	Swelling								
	Fitness								
Week 4	Pain								
	Stiffness								
	Swelling								
	Fitness								

For this monthly tracker, I recommend using 1-3 for level of pain or stiffness and + or − for fitness activity. The number 1 should be designated as little or tolerable pain or swelling and 3 as severe. Our goal is for average pain or swelling of 1 and six "+" days for fitness activity.

10 Pounds are 10 years

The effect of our weight on our joints is undeniable. Obesity itself is a risk for the development of OA. It has been found that 1 pound of weight gain has a four pound effect on the stress of the knee in walking. Losing 10 pounds should, therefore, offer a great relief for your knees and hips. I like to say "10 pounds are like 10 years." That is, your legs will feel years younger by losing 10 pounds. You can do this.

Exercise, as it turns out, is an inefficient way to lose weight. An average person walking briskly for 30 minutes may burn about 100 calories. Not much, is it? Besides, vigorous exercise tends to stimulate our appetites as our body recovers from the change in activity and prepares for more activity. Routine exercise may help to burn energy and achieve our goals, but just think about how much walking you would have to do to lose 1 pound of fat; 3500 calories. It turns out that gentle diet restriction is more effective at weight loss than is exercise alone. I would, of course, recommend both diet and exercise because we cannot be healthy if we do not exercise, and the weight lost in dieting is best maintained by routine exercise.

Do not be discouraged by failed attempts at weight loss. We are destined to gain weight. Think of our recent and distant ancestors. Our bodies have evolved to survive periods of want or famine. When we eat or are inactive, our bodies efficiently store energy in complex sugars and fats and even tear down inactive muscle to conserve energy. Combine this energy storage with our appetite and it is no wonder that we all tend to gain weight with time. Our brains, fat cells and even our stomachs have appetite signals that make us want to eat, even when we are not hungry. Our appetites become even stronger when we use starvation as a way to lose weight. And when we starve ourselves, our metabolism slows making weight loss more difficult.

You will have a healthy weight if you exercise well and eat well. It may not be what you want when you look in the mirror. But that is another issue. If you want to look thin it takes even greater effort. First, go for a healthy weight with an initial 10 pound loss to protect your arthritic joints.

Before you start a diet program, review your previous diet experience. Look at your past successes with weight loss. Was it on your own or with other people? What happened to make you stop your successful approach? Look also at your mistakes. Did starvation diets or temporary diets guarantee that you would regain your lost weight? Did you tell others that you were on a diet but lived as if you had no plan? Consider what you have learned and develop a plan for healthy weight loss. Use this new plan everyday. Incorporate what you have learned from past experience. Plan now to forgive yourself for bad days since some are inevitable. If you can make most days good days, you will lose weight. If you can reduce your calories by 100 each day, you will lose those 10 pounds in one year—without a doubt. If you exercise 100 calories worth daily and cut back by 100 calories (about a slice of bread) a day you can count on 20 pounds of weight loss in one year. Decreasing the amount of carbohydrates in your diet (breads, cereals, rice, pasta and potatoes) while maintaining healthy vegetable, fruit, and protein intake is probably the easiest and most effective diet technique.

We usually trick ourselves by splurging on occasion. We may have many good diet days and when a party or other event arises we forget that we have a plan. Sometimes we even trick ourselves into thinking that if we have six good days we can have one bad day. This usually will not work if we have modest calorie losses, one piece of cake or a sugary coffee drink may more than make up for the previous week's calorie loss.

When it comes to specific diet approaches I recommend those that you can follow for a lifetime and that have no apparent hazard. The diet plans I typically recommend in my clinic are Weight Watchers, South Beach, or the Ornish diet. For those who benefit from shared goals and working with others Weight Watchers is a good place to start a weight loss program. For those who can make and stick to meal plans without outside support, the South Beach Diet is a reasonable and healthy diet plan. For those who cannot or will not consider low carbohydrate diets follow the Ornish diet. Each of the above plans will help with weight loss and lessen the risks of diabetes and cardiovascular disease. There are other plans that work as well, just check with a health professional if you are uncertain about the use or potential pitfalls of other diet plans. Please note that I do not receive support from these or any of the commercial products mentioned in this book.

When the weight loss reaches ten pounds it is ok to eat a little bit more, but be careful. Maintain near daily activity and weigh yourself on a good scale daily to help maintain the weight loss. Once you feel the difference in your joints, you may want to plan additional weight loss. If you are uncertain about how much loss is needed, please ask your physician or nutritionist. In general, if a person is obese or overweight a ten-percent weight loss will reduce or eliminate the severity of many of the weight-related diseases such as high blood pressure or diabetes. Please aim first for health and accept the results you work for. If you then want to shape your body in a certain way or have a specific "thin" weight you want to achieve, go for it. Remember that we sometimes fail in our diet and weight loss due to unrealistic expectations of body shape or sex-appeal. When we do not find the attention we expected we will return to the unhealthy lifestyle that brought us to overweight or obesity. Keep in mind, there is not one "sexy" body type and "sexy" is not just what others determine for us. For example, it has been proven that active overweight women with small amounts of weight loss can enjoy a much-improved sex life and sense of attractiveness. So go for health and enjoy the benefits that a little weight loss can bring. Even a "fit arthritic" can be satisfied with moderate weight loss and improved sense of attractiveness.

Exercise for Your Life

Exercise is essential for good health, especially joint or heart health. It is unfortunate that exercise or sports, especially with injury may have contributed to our joint disease. Mine started from competitive volleyball. I played in tournaments that lasted hours, playing when I was tired, injured and not always in proper condition. When it was clear that I should have stopped, I tried to continue playing, taking too many aspirin and ibuprofen, before I quit for good. I eventually had to give up on even friendly volleyball games in the park or on company picnics. Bicycling was beneficial for my knees but the outcome was so good I tried running again to supplement my exercise routine. This started causing pain and swelling in my one damaged knee and soon led to discouragement. I stuck with cycling for a while and then tried to play tennis with my wife, with only painful results. My doctor told me not to play tennis, but really had no other words of advice. The surgeon for my first damaged knee had not explained how I had a condition that would place me at risk of joint degeneration and pain. If I had advanced warning, I may have spent more time in beneficial activity and reduced my time in damaging activity.

A later surgery on the previously "good" knee slowed me down. I was more discouraged. A minor injury led to an arthroscopic (joint camera) surgery that revealed serious articular cartilage damage to the knee that had given me no symptoms prior to the injury. After having this surgery, I spent some time in the gym and some on a bicycle but I did not get anywhere except more out of shape, weaker in my legs and with more pain. If only I knew then what I know now! I would not have gained 70 pounds and spent so much time in pain or waste money on medication that did not help my joints.

I encourage the use of an arthritis diary. You can use the format I suggest in the chapter on pain and its treatment. Use a scale of 1 to 3, 1 to 10, or good to bad to describe pain and stiffness and swelling. If every week the pain and stiffness increases and fitness in not increasing it is time to reassess your activity. Please elicit help from your physical therapist, physician, sports medicine physician or orthopedic specialist. Use the pain and stiffness score to compare to your fitness goals to determine your progress.

Exercise includes aerobic movement (walking and cycling are examples), stretching (such as yoga) and strengthening. Strengthening exercise may be isometric (no movement) or with movement (isotonic or dynamic). Isotonic exercise uses fixed weight or resistance and dynamic exercise uses resistance bands/rods or machines to change the resistance (weight) throughout the range of the exercise. These are simplifications since the benefits of exercise overlap. For example, yoga will strengthen as it stretches and cycling will strengthen the leg muscles as well. Yoga or Tai Chi are wonderful forms of exercise and may supplement aerobic exercise in our management of our joint disease. I will not emphasize stretches in the exercise regimen, but I support your effort to explore these forms of movement and would like to hear about your results.

For those with knee arthritis it is most important to strengthen the quadriceps muscle ("quads" as they are often called). The quads are the muscles in the front on the thigh that make the lower leg move forward. They are the muscles that support us in a squat position. The gluteus muscles ("glutes") are the muscles most compromised in OA of the hip and therefore the muscles most likely to offer relief and stability when exercised. The glutes are actually three muscles that form the outline of our buttocks and help us in sitting or arising and in climbing stairs. Remember, the muscles around the OA-affected joints tend to waste and weaken due to the pain that result in reflex relaxation signals from the spinal cord. Since I have two knees (and one hip, wrist, hand, and my neck) with OA and one knee is more affected than the other, the most affected leg is thinner than the other and remains so even with regular exercise. The reflex weakening of the major muscles around the joints causes further instability of the joint and this instability from weakness puts us at greater risk of OA with minimal use of the joint. This is why avoiding exercise is not a good option since our joints are going to weaken, destabilize and wear with minimal use. Not only that, we will then gain weight which will also wear our joints. So exercising our diseased joints maintains muscle strength and size and protects the joint from instability.

Jarring of our joints is to be avoided. This makes running, especially running on concrete prohibited with OA. The primary aerobic exercise should be cycling for OA of the knees or hips. I believe that a recumbent cycle or exerciser is even better than an upright cycle. I own a recumbent indoor exerciser and a traditional bicycle. If you are buying a bicycle or exerciser, be sure to purchase your machine from someone who can help you fit the bicycle/machine and help you adjust it for best use. In general, your legs should be nearly straight with the toes slightly flexed downward when the cycle's pedal is at its farthest position. For an upright cycle, it is ideal also for your knee to be straight above the ball of your foot when the pedal is midway down. Please see the photo in the exercise section demonstrating proper leg position.

Walking is probably ok for most with OA. I recommend wearing well-padded walking or running shoes for walking and everyday activity. There are newly designed shoes for OA of the knee, but are not readily available so I will not go into detail about them in this edition of this book. Walking should be smooth and not jarring of the joints. Some of us may benefit from special braces or knee wraps, please check with your OA specialist (physical therapist, physician or orthopedist) regarding your use of braces. If you need a cane or walker, be sure to ask for instruction on their proper use. I notice that the slight angle of the sidewalks and roadways may stress my joints so I make sure to spend equal time on opposite sides to minimize discomfort.

Strengthening exercise protects and stabilizes the joint and allows for the aerobic exercise that helps to prevent or delay the age-related diseases of heart attack/ stroke, dementia, osteoporosis and falls. Strengthening should emphasize the large protective muscle groups, but will also involve all of the muscles in our hips and legs. The calf and posterior thigh muscles also contribute to knee stability and hip flexor and front thigh muscles will contribute to hip stability.

Exercises for the Knee

Strengthening Exercises for the Knee

In the chapter "Achieving Fitness" I described how to start an aerobic conditioning program. Strengthening exercise also rehabilitates osteoarthritis joints. I recommend starting a strengthening program on an every other day basis. Once your strength is where you want it these exercises can then be performed once or twice a week. With time you will get a feel of how often to do these exercises and may notice improvement in pain and stiffness on the days that you do them. Do not be discouraged if there is some pain and swelling after starting these exercises. Review the exercises with your OA specialist to verify which exercises you may do. Some of these exercises can be done daily. For example if my knee starts to hurt, I will often extend my leg, tighten my quads and hold it for multiple 10-15 second repetitions. This often provides immediate relief and helps my knee feel more stable as I am walking on those painful days.

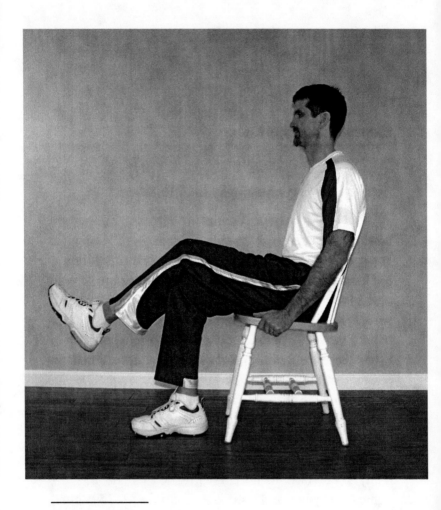

Knee Extension

In a seated position hold your foot straight out. In small movements let your knee bend then tighten your quads again to straighten the leg again. Perform 10-15 repetitions (reps) or hold for 10-15 seconds for 3-5 reps. The long-term goal is to perform 3 or more sets of these repetitions. Do not do this at the gym on the leg extension machines unless you have been cleared to do so by your arthritis specialist.

Knee Extension with Resistance

Same as knee extension except these are done with weights, such as light ankle weights. I do this exercise for pain relief on my stiff and achy days.

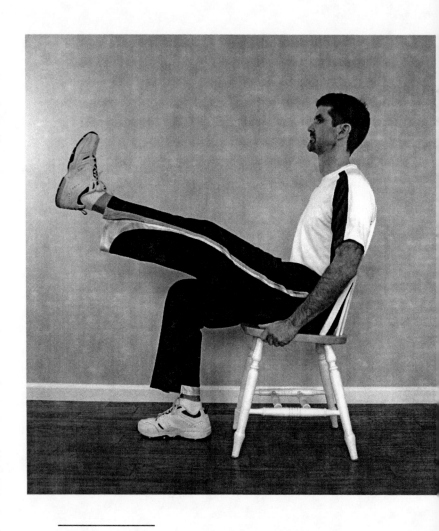

Leg lifts

The Leg lift is similar to knee extension, except that the leg is straight and the entire leg is lifted at the hip. Perform 10-15 reps with a goal of 3 or more sets.

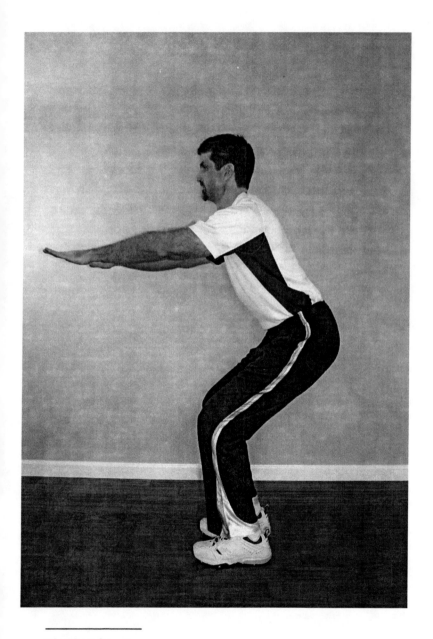

Modified Squat

Modified Squat

The squat is a simple exercise that uses all of our lower body muscles. For arthritis be sure to move your behind backward ("butt-back") so that your knees remain over and not in front of your feet. Start with limited motion and increase your range over time so that your knees approach a maximum of 90 degrees of flexion. You may increase the challenge by holding weights in your hands. Start with 5-10 repetitions with a goal of 3 sets. Do not hold a squat position when exercising your arthritic knees.

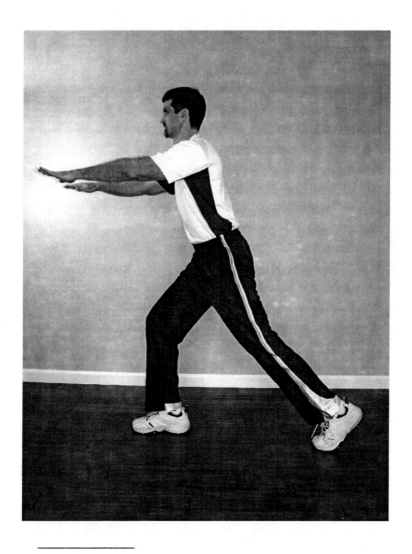

Modified One-Legged Squat, the Reverse Lunge

The Reverse Lunge

This exercise will increase the strength throughout the leg. Perform this exercise by lifting the opposite foot and placing it behind you while squatting with one leg. Then lift the leg again and use your bent leg to return to a standing position. Your knee should be directly over the ball of your foot when the knee is bent. Holding weights in your hands will increase the challenge for this exercise as well. Leaning the body forward (while maintaining a straight back) will increase the use of the glutes. I use this variation to simulate hiking uphill. Start with 5-10 reps with a goal of 3 sets. Limit the amount of knee bend initially and do not bend the knee more than 90 degrees even when you are stronger and more advanced.

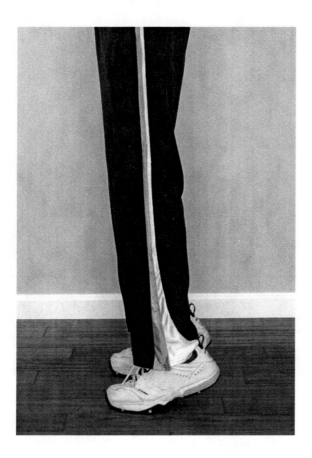

Calf raises

The calf muscles cross the knee joint and add to its stability. You may do these one at a time or together. For more challenge these can be done on a step, allowing the heel to drop slightly below the ball of the foot. Start with 10-20 reps with a goal of 3 sets.

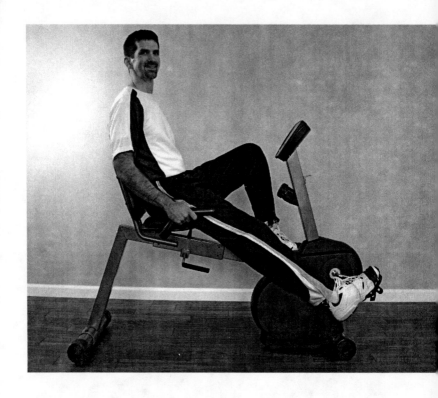

Cycling

When cycling, the leg should be nearly straight with the ball of the foot downward on the down stroke. On the up stroke the knees should be comfortably flexed. In mid-down stroke the knee should be over the toes. Cycling or walking can be enjoyed daily. Start with five minutes once daily. You may add a minute each time and have multiple sessions per day. Three ten minutes episodes of aerobic activity (walking or cycling) are at least as valuable as one thirty minute session.

Strengthening exercises for the Hip

Leg Lift

See leg lift in the exercises for the knee.

Leg Lift with Lateral Movement

Same as leg lift, except that the straight leg is held slightly outward from the body.

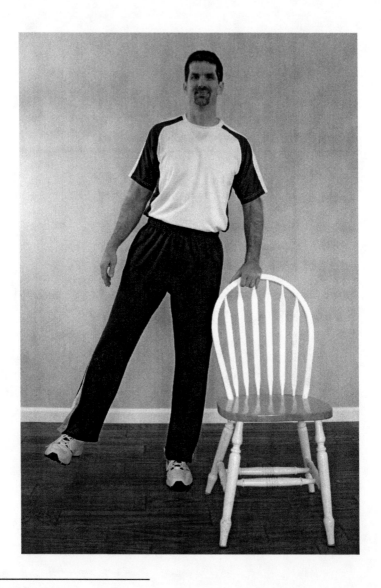

Leg Abduction

This may be done standing or lying on your side. Move the leg out and relax in. Start with 10-20 reps with a goal of 3 sets.

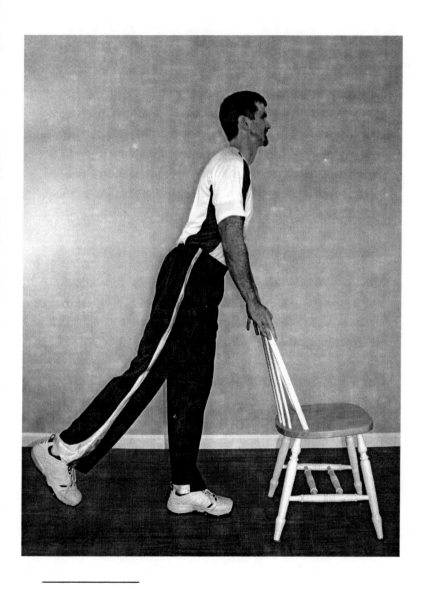

Gluteus Extension

Gluteus Extension

This may be done standing erect or leaning forward. It may be done from hands-and-knees position but for my arthritic patients I usually do not recommend it. Move your leg backwards as far as is comfortable and relax to the starting position. Start with 10-20 reps with a goal of 3 sets. Ankle weights will increase the challenge when you are ready.

Gluteus Extension with External Rotation

This will challenge the lateral glutes by rotating your foot outward and then extending the leg behind you. This may be done in addition to the extension with similar recommendations for reps and sets.

Modified Squat and Reverse Lunge

These exercises are reviewed under knee exercises.

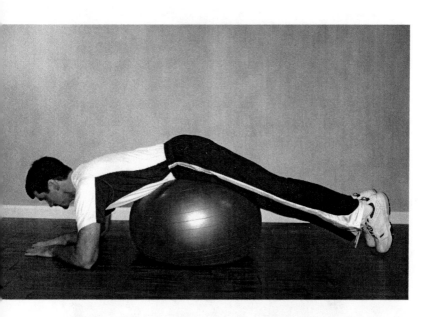

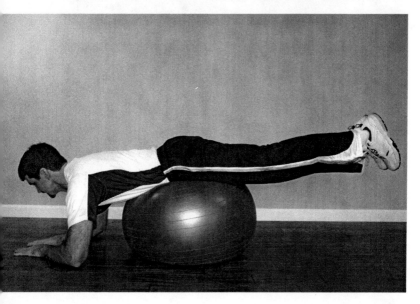

Ball Extension

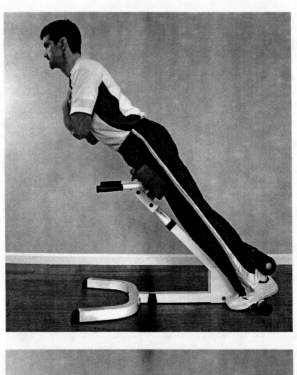

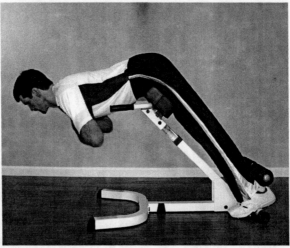

Roman Chair Extension

Ball and Roman Chair Extension

This exercise will use all of the muscles of the back of the leg and include some of the muscles of the low and middle back. One or both legs are lifted off the ground while the upper body is stabilized over an exercise ball. Alternatively, at the gym the legs are held in place while the upper body is lowered and raised in the "roman chair." Please ask for instruction if you plan to use the roman chair at the gym.

Cycling

Cycling provides motion and strengthening of the entire hip without impact. If an upright cycle or standard bicycle is uncomfortable, try a recumbent exercise cycle. I even recommend this exercise to my patients that are awaiting a hip replacement. Most of these patients find a recumbent exercise cycle surprisingly easy.

After word

My purpose in writing this book is to encourage you to seek health and show you some of the ways that you may become strong and fit with OA. I wish you well in your pursuit of good health. I do recommend that you use my book along with the support of a good physical therapist or physician. I cannot guarantee that you will become fit and avoid a joint replacement, but I am confident that you will not have your expert disagree with my overall message. I have reviewed the scientific literature and have applied what I found to myself and I am enjoying less disability 20 years after the start of the disease process. I am confident that proper exercise and activity performs better than any medication or supplements. Most physicians will treat the pain (with medication) but not have the time to help us prepare for the future of OA. I hope that my book helps you and your physician prepare for the future. Unfortunately, I cannot include everything I know into one book. I am unable in this book to discuss some of the nuances of OA and its treatments. I have not mentioned partial joint replacement, hyaluronate injections, specialized braces, footwear and other treatment options that may benefit some of us. I have not discussed the issue of timing of joint replacement in this book either. These types of issues I would expect your expert to discuss with you. I believe that my book will help your specialist spend better quality of time individualizing treatment for you if you use this as a guide to fitness with OA. I am writing about many of the things that I should have known early in my struggle with OA. Please let me know how you are doing.

Wishing you the best of health,

Alan Kelton M.D.
The Fit Arthritic

P.S. I do recognize that referring to a person by their disease state can seem insensitive. I personally have no problem with the term "arthritic" to describe my physical being since daily I am limited by the condition. I cannot even jog across the street to beat a quick walk signal without risking days to weeks of pain and stiffness—that is "arthritic." Yet I do have some sense of accomplishment in that I can match many healthy men my age in strength and endurance. If you have taken offense to the use of the term "arthritic," I am sorry. Please recognize that there are many of us who will use the term to describe ourselves without such concern and will use the term with pride.

Resources

The Fit Arthritic: www.fitarthritic.com

Arthritis Foundation: www.arthritis.org

LaVergne, TN USA
23 August 2009
155651LV00001B/66/P